R e i k i

The First Degree

By

Antje Ursula Seebohm

Reiki

The First Degree

©Antje Ursula Seebohm

Malta 2012

For Pete in Love and Gratitude.
You are the Light of my Life!

Table of Contents

About the Author

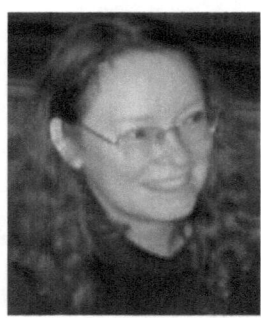

Antje Ursula Seebohm

was born in Hamburg/Germany in 1956. After working as a lawyer for an insurance company for more than 20 years without really being happy with that career, she decided to give her life a completely new direction.

In July 2006 she made the decision to move to Malta together with her second husband Peter, where she has been living and working ever since.

Antje received her first Reiki attunement in 2001. After that almost 3 years passed during which she did not feel the need to go on with Reiki.

It was only in 2004 when suddenly she felt the urge to attend a Reiki 2 class, and then immediately proceeded to Master/Teacher that same year.

Since then she has successfully attuned a number of clients to all Reiki Degrees, including a few distance attunements.

In Dec 2008 she has also been certified as a Clinical Hypnotherapist.

What is Reiki?

Reiki is a simple hands-on technique for transferring energy.

It's simple because you receive the ability to transfer the energy passively through an attunement. So you don't have to study, meditate or exercise for years.

Of course you will need a bit of know-how to work with Reiki. But this can be learnt within a few hours.

The term Reiki (pronounced Ray Key) comes from the Japanese language. „Rei" means „The Universe", and „Ki" means „life force" (that same vital energy whose existence is acknowledged in any culture, whether it's called „Chi" in China, „Prana" in India or „Lebenskraft" in Germany – just as a few examples).

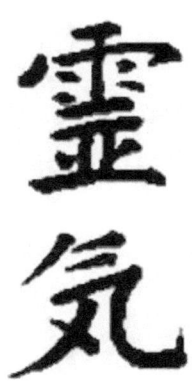

So for once Reiki is the universal life force that surrounds us everywhere.

However the expression Reiki is not only used for this force itself, but also for the way to handle it, which means that Reiki also names the ability to draw vital energy from our surroundings and pass it on to others (or to ourselves) in order to harmonize and energize them.

Basically this is an ability that we all have by nature. But most of us have lost it due to our hectic modern lifestyle. The Reiki attunements clear the energy channels and reinstate this natural ability.

The attunements work for everybody – though of course you must be aware that there will always be differences in the intensity and quality of the energy flow. Everybody can sing, but some people's voices sound like there's an angel singing, whilst others rather remind you of an alarm signal. And every (healthy) body can run or swim, but not everyone is going to break a world record. Practice helps here as everywhere – the more you use Reiki, the more you integrate it into your life, the stronger it gets!

A Reiki practitioner does not give away his own energy. He only channels the energy, and as it runs through him before it reaches the recipient he usually feels better after a treatment too.

Anyone who has received a proper attunement is able to transfer the energy spontaneously, without any special concentration, meditation or prayer. It's the intention that counts. You just decide you want the energy to flow, and it does! Therefore a practitioner can provide himself or a third person with the energy instantly, without having to carry any tools on him. You always have your hands on you!

Usually this effect of an attunement is permanent. Even though I've heard of people who lost their ability after going through situations that caused them extreme stress over a significant period of time, such as getting injured in a heavy accident, going through a painful divorce or similar circumstances.

The best you can do to keep your channels open no matter what is to keep on using Reiki! However I'm always offering my students to re-attune them free of charge should they ever feel the need for this. Up to now nobody has approached me for that reason!

Reiki benefits humans, animals, plants – and sometimes it even works for things such as machines, batteries, computers etc.. Reiki permeates each and every material, clothes, casts, braces, metal and concrete. Reiki can be applied in any situation. It harmonizes and helps restore the balance between body, spirit and soul.

Usually Reiki is taught in 3 or 4 Degrees, but there could be more or less, depending on the system that the Master is following.

The Reiki 1 Degree opens the Reiki channels and enables the student to transfer the energy through his hands to himself or others. However the recipient needs to be present so the practitioner can actually put his hands on him.

During the Reiki 2 Class three Reiki Symbols are introduced to the student. The First Symbol helps him boost the energy flow. The Second Symbol provides him with a key to the unconscious mind to help him perform mental healings. And the Third Symbol enables the practitioner to bridge time and space, so he can send Reiki either to another person who is not present (Distance or Remote Reiki) or into his own past or future (Situation Healing) .

During the Reiki 3 Class (Master/Teacher Degree) the student is attuned to the Master Symbol and learns how to use it in meditation. He also learns how to teach Reiki and how to attune students to the different levels of Reiki himself.

However many students want the Master Degree for their own benefit only, in order to raise their own vibrational energy, but have no intention to ever teach others. Like many other teachers I have therefore decided to offer Reiki 3A (Master Degree only) and 3B (Teacher) Classes. This makes the Master Degree affordable for everyone.

This e-book deals with the First Degree only, but Volumes 2 and 3 are soon to follow.

How does Reiki work?

Everything is Energy

Even objects that appear quite solid, such as a table or a wall, aren't as solid as they seem. You could actually see that if you cut out a piece and put it under a microscope that's strong enough to bring it down to the smallest unit.

Every object consists of molecules that are built of atoms. The chemical formula for water for example is H_2O, which means that water molecules consist of 2 atoms of hydrogen and 1 atom of oxygen. And under your very strong microscope you could see that there is indeed a lot of space between those atoms.

When I was a child scientists thought that atoms are the smallest existing unit. But then Quantumphysics evolved, and found out that the atoms themselves are built of protons, neutrons and electrons, which again consist of quarks.

Scientific tests on quarks later showed that these aren't really particles, but „entities of energy" that behave like waves rather than objects.

But I'm not a scientist and I don't want to go further into this topic. I hope you can agree to the basic concept that brought down to the smallest unit known to us so far everything is basically the same: Energy.

Because all that I said applies not only to non-organic matter such as objects, liquids or gas, but to living beings - humans, animals and plants - as well.

The mystery is what determines that a table is perceived as a table, and a person like you and me as a person. There are different concepts in Quantumphysics about that too, and it's probably consciousness – but again we don't have to dig deeper into this.

The Human Energy System

So what you and I need to know, is that basically everything – and everyone - consists of the same energy. This energy is not static, it's vibrating and pulsating.

If you look at an acupuncture chart, you will see a variety of lines that run all over the human body, the so-called energy meridians.

The following picture shows an ancient Chinese acupuncture chart from the Ming Dynasty:

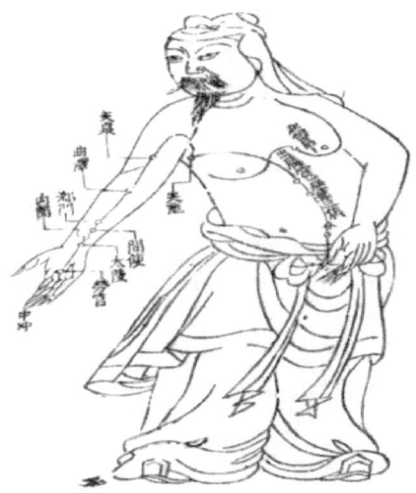

As you can see this ancient chart is is not very detailed. The modern ones that you'll find on the internet if you google „Acupuncture chart" are a lot more complicated and look like expansive traffic maps. And in a way that's what they are, as they show the routes on which the electricity travels along our our bodies.

Many of those meridians end on the soles of our feet, but also on our hands and ears. That explains why a massage on the feet and hands – reflexology – can have such a profound effect on remote areas of our bodies. What not so many people know is that reflexology on the ears is even more effective, but it sure makes sense if you consider that the skin on the ears is extremely delicate compared to that on our feet.

Then there are 7 main energetic centers in our body, the Chakras (which means wheel or vortex). The Chakras are aligned along the spine from bottom to top and the correspondent areas on the front of the body. They draw energy from the environment and redistribute it, thus feeding our energy field, the so-called „aura".

There are specific colours that correspond to each Chakra, and different body parts as well as typical issues are attributed to them, which means that if a Chakra doesn't function properly you might experience problems in the respective area, either on the physical or on the mental/emotional side.

For details see the following table:

	Name	Location	Colour	Associated Body Parts	Issues
Seventh Chakra	Crown Chakra	Top of the Head	violet	Upper Skull, Cerebral Cortex, Skin	Spirituality, Connection to Higher Source
Sixth Chakra	Third Eye Chakra	Between and above the Eyebrows	indigo	Eyes, Sinuses, Base of Skull, Temporal Lobes	Intuition, Trust
Fifth Chakra	Throat Chakra	Throat Area	sky blue	Throat, Mouth, Teeth, Jaw, Ears	Communication Speaking Your Truth, Self-Expression
Fourth Chakra	Heart Chakra	Chest Area	green	Pericardium, Heart, Lungs, Circulation	Balance, Loving Yourself and Others
Third Chakra	Solar Plexus Chakra	Above the Navel	yellow	Stomach, Liver, Gall Bladder, Pancreas, Small Intestine, Muscles	Personal Power, Confidence, Self-Esteem
Second Chakra	Sacral Chakra	Lower Abdomen	orange	Sex Organs, Bladder, Uterus or Prostate	Feelings and Emotions, Joy, Sexuality, Creativity
First Chakra	Root Chakra	Base of the Spine	red	Kidneys, Blood and Skeletal System	Grounding, Safety, Physical Existence, Wealth

Most cultures agree on the 7 main Chakras that are mentioned above. However there are a few cultures, the Native Americans for example, who speak of 8 Chakras. The 8th Chakra is located about 10 cm above your head and is another connection to God or Higher Source, how ever you want to call Him (or Her).

Whilst in past times the existence of the Chakras was

nothing but a concept, today their frequencies can actually be measured, and the aura of a person, which shines in an individual mix of the colors above, can be made visible with Kirlian-Photography (a specific photographic technique, accidentally developed by Semyon Kirlian in 1939 and later refined by others).

Every thing and every person have their own specific vibration. (By the way this also applies to the thoughts and feelings that you produce during the day, and that you send out into the universe just like radio waves.)

If the energy field of a person is intact, and all the Chakras are open so the life force „Ki" flows freely and without blockages, he is physically and mentally healthy.

But sometimes the flow of the energy is blocked. This may have relatively simple causes. Just sitting in front of a computer in an unhealthy posture day-in and day-out until the muscles are so tight that they don't even relax over night can be enough. In fact the reason can be anything: from ongoing stress, unhealthy eating habits, sleep disorders, via infections, injury, mental traumata, up to misuse of alcohol or drugs.

If the situation persists, this may lead to serious disease. Therefore the blockages must be broken and the energy flow enforced.

And that's what a treatment with Reiki does.

Like other energy healing techniques, Reiki is a

holistic treatment. Most Reiki practitioners are no medical doctors, so we never diagnose. And actually we don't necessarily need to know what the problem is and if it has a name, as we don't treat a disease. All a Reiki practitioner can do is provide the client with extra energy. If and how the recipient uses it is up to him. But this may be just the one „Kick" the client needs to turn the situation around and have his body heal itself.

Of course the results depend on the strength of the blockage and the damage that's already been done to the body, as well as on the constancy and intensity of the Reiki treatments.

Treatments with Reiki have often caused spontaneous healing. However some recipients unconsciously resist the energy. You never know the hidden reason why somebody suffers from a certain disease. It may even be part of his karmic development. Therefore results can and must never be promised or even guaranteed!

But this does NOT mean that the healing power of Reiki should be underestimated!

Whenever I give Reiki to someone I try to detach myself completely from the outcome, as I know that it's not me who is doing the healing anyway, but the client himself.

So usually I tell the client to just be open, let the energy work and then see what happens. And often enough even I have been surprised by what's possible!

Just one example: I've had a client who was suffering from chronic back pain. There was some part in his lower back that would lock in and cause him heavy pain whenever he got up from a chair or his bed. He had tried about everything, and the doctors in hospital had told him there was nothing they could do for him, so he would have to live with that pain.
When he approached me I really had doubts that Reiki could do much in this case, and as it's not my style to make promises that I can't keep I was quite open about this. I told him that if the problem was on the mechanical side then Reiki surely couldn't change this. But what it could do was relax him and thus relieve some of the pain and the stress he was going through.

He decided to try it anyway. And after the treatment at least he got up from the bench without pain. My husband who was just returning from shopping saw him walk away and told me that this client was now moving like a different person, with much more ease and energy than when he came.

So far so good. However I didn't hear again from this client, so I thought that it probably hadn't worked out that well for him. Then after almost 2 years I received an email which read:

„Hi Antje,

I have been for reiki session(was suffering from back pain) at your

previous address and I must say felt the benefit immediately, I
thoroughly recommend Reiki technique.
I would appreciate if you could advise whether it's possible to make
an appointment for my wife who at present is suffering from neck pain ..."

I was completely blown away when I read this because I really hadn't expected it in this specific case!

He wrote „ ... **was** suffering from back pain ...". So that one session that he had with me actually helped him get rid of this!!!

Of course I'm not getting feedback from every client, but from what I've heard it's not an exception that clients get healed after only one treatment. Sometimes I receive an email the next day, or a few days after the treatment, letting me know that they are fine!

What I've actually noticed is that the healing power of my sessions is increasing more and more with practice. And I'm truly happy about this. Reiki is my passion, I love and respect every one of my clients, and it's just good to know that I really am of service to them!!!

But don't get me wrong. I am by no means a „Wonder Healer" and never claimed to be. Up to now I haven't had a client here with a potentially terminal disease such as cancer, but some time ago I treated a friend in Germany as well as one of my aunts who lived in Paris with Distance Reiki. They both suffered from cancer, which was already quite advanced when I learnt about it, and unfortunately they both died.

If the recipient is very ill it may indeed happen that even though Reiki removes the blockages and reinstates a healthy flow of energy, the damages in the body are too grave already to be repaired.

And of course we have to accept that we're not immortal anyway, so everyone of us will go when our time has come.

This explains why a patient may die even though he receives regular Reiki treatments. But he is still going to benefit from the sessions as they help him accept what's happening, take away some of the pain he may experience and actually ease the transition.

Please note: If the client has a condition, always ask him to see his doctor or medical practitioner for approval first.

It should be understood that the client must never stop to take any prescribed medication.

Reiki is a complementary rather than an alternative treatment. And it's greatest benefit lies in the field of prevention, so the client doesn't get sick in the first place!

A Short History of Reiki

Usually I don't like to dig too deeply into the history of Reiki. Most of it is a myth anyway ...

But of course there are some basics that the student should know.

The popular healing system that most people know as Reiki today was founded by **Dr. Mikao Usui**, who lived in Japan and died in 1926 at the age of 62.

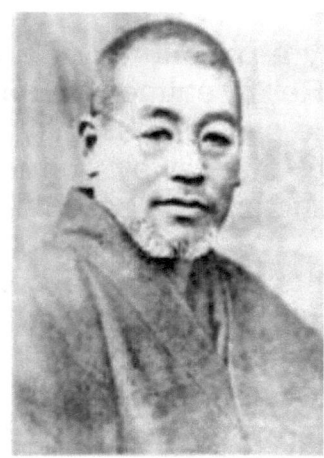

Unfortunately there are hardly any facts confirmed about his life.

It's quite certain that he wasn't a Doctor of Medicine. Some people speculate that he must have been some high administration official as he had the possibility to travel and obviously had access to secret documents too. Others say that he was a Japanese born Christian monk. However it's not confirmed that he really was Christian, and this may have been said in order to make Reiki more acceptable for the US-American market.

Whatever the truth is, he did have a successful healing practice later in his life.

There are many legends about how or why he found the 4 Symbols that later made the foundation of the Usui Reiki System. What is known is that in the beginning of his healing practice no „Symbols" were used. But after Usui noticed at some point that his students had great difficulties in maintaining the level of concentration that's necessary if you want to perform an energy transfer without using any tools, he started searching for a solution.

One legend says that one day he was asked by a student how Jesus used to heal. He could not answer this question, but it never left him alone and so he tried to find out. And even though he never found the answer, instead he found the way in which The Buddha healed - Reiki!

Another legend says that the Symbols were actually revealed to him on the last night of a 21-day retreat in the mountains where he was attuned by the Higher Power itself. At first he didn't realize what had happened, but on his long way back home a few incidents occured that made him aware of his new healing powers.

Whether it really happened that way, or whether he studied some ancient scripts, the truth doesn't really matter. Somehow he did discover (or rather re-discover) those Symbols and their healing power, and he spent the rest of his life performing healing treatments and teaching Reiki all over Japan.

By the way: Dr. Usui wasn't the only one who discovered those „Symbols". I know of at least one alternative Reiki-System, founded by a Tibetan Monk of French origin by the name of Serge Goldberg and later taught by Oswald Wirth. Goldberg re-discovered exactly the same 4 Symbols that Dr. Usui used at about the same time (strange synchronicities like this happen again and again in history).

Even though their Reiki system is given away for free, most people never heard of Serge Goldberg and Oswald Wirth. Maybe it's just a question of marketing. Or maybe it's because they hardly gave instructions on how to actually use the Symbols (at least as far as I've been told by someone who attended a seminar with Oswald Wirth). Most beginners want clear directions – this definitely applied to me when I first started with Reiki.

But back to Dr. Usui: after he became aware that most diseases don't have only physical reasons he added some rules for life to his system of Reiki healing:

Just for Today Do not worry, Accept
Just for today, do not anger.
Honour your parents, teachers and elders
Earn your living honestly
Show gratitude to all living things.

The system of the 3 Degrees was not in place at that time, but Dr. Usui used to give what later was called the First Degree to anyone who needed and wanted it and the Second Degree to only a few, mostly people who worked for him. But only to sixteen of his students he revealed the Fourth or Master Symbol which allows you to initiate other people.

One of them was **Dr. Chujiro Hayashi**

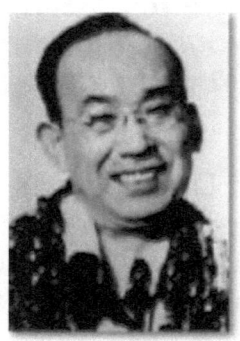

who continued to develop the Usui System of healing in his own health clinic in Tokyo after Usui's death. Dr. Hayashi carefully took note of the techniques that were most successfully used in his clinic and introduced the standard hand positions. He also created the Three Degree System and their initiation procedures.

Dr. Hayashi initiated 13 Reiki Masters. The last one of them was Mrs. **Hawayo Takata**.

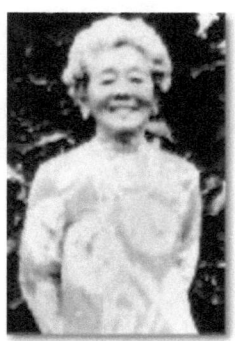

Mrs. Takata was a Hawaiian-born American of Japanese origin.

She went to Japan to find healing from different serious conditions. After she was healed in Dr. Hayashi's clinic in Tokyo she became his student. Later Mrs. Takata brought Reiki back to the United States and founded a health clinic in Hawaii. She also made Reiki a commercial system and became very prosperous.

Mrs. Takata only started to initiate other masters when she was already in her seventies. She initiated 22 masters.

At that time she used to charge 10,000 USD for the Master/Teacher Degree!

Some Reiki organisations still stick to this rate. But even though relatively seen 10,000 USD are not the same today as they used to be then, I still find that price a bit exaggerated. Many Reiki Masters see it that way too, so today the cost can be significantly lower for you if you choose an independent Reiki Master.

This may be one of the reasons why Reiki has spread all over the world.

After the death of Mrs. Takata in 1980 Reiki split into several directions. Unfortunately some of them severely oppose each other, each one claiming "The true Reiki" for themselves. This sure is not in the sense of Reiki which represents love and harmony and peaceful co-existence!

Some strictly follow the original system that Dr. Usui and Dr. Hayashi founded. Others have made modifications to the original system, and up to 20 new "Grand Master" Degrees have been added (maybe even more as I write this).

You have to decide for yourself if this really is for the better ...

I'm not of the opinion that things have to remain unchanged always and forever. Change is a natural thing, and often a very positive one. All things have to expand and grow.

I myself was curious, so I explored a few additional Degrees (up to the 12th) and alternative Reiki Systems such as Inti-Reiki and Trinitas „the Christian Reiki". I even purchased the exclusive rights to teach Trinitas here in Malta.

However as it turned out I don't really use them.

In my practice I have found that the original Usui Reiki-System offers everything that you really need. So this is what I'm teaching today. However I have implied a few minor changes into my personal practice that made more sense to me.

All the same I always encourage my students to think for themselves and to find out what's right for them!

How to work with Reiki

Reiki is simple and doesn't need a lot of preparation or rules. It can be applied at any time and in any possible place. As I said: You always have your hands on you!

Still there are some recommendations that are meant to even enhance the well-being of the recipient.

Please note: even if none of them are followed, Reiki still flows. The only real condition is that the practitioner must have had a proper attunement.

And of course he must intend to give Reiki.

The following recommendations are useful, but optional:

Place:
Reiki can be used anywhere. But to make the recipient relax best you should go to a light, quiet room if you can. If you don't have a professional Reiki bench the recipient could lie on a couch or a blanket on the floor.

But keep your own well-being in mind! This low position could be very uncomfortable for your own back! And you can't really be a perfect open channel if you suffer from back pain!

So if you plan on doing treatments regularly, it would be wise to invest in a simple bench (you can sometimes find used ones on eBay that aren't too expensive).

There is also a Short Treatment with the recipient sitting that I'm going to teach you. If you don't have a bench you will probably apply this more often than the regular treatment. But of course the recipient won't relax as much as he does when he lies down. Also some of the positions are quite intimate as you'll get very close. So I recommend this for use with close friends or family only, not for professional treatments.

Clothing:
Both the practitioner as well as the recipient can wear whatever they want. But it would be wise to choose something comfortable, in which you can move freely and that you won't ruin when you lie down!

Music:
This is optional. I use New Age Music that's specially been composed for Reiki Treatments. Some pieces have a little bell ringing after either 3 or 5 minutes, which is a nice reminder for changing the hand position.

Scent:
Of course you could do without it. I evaporate relaxing essential oils such as Neroli, Lavender or Sandalwood (but ask the recipient in case he's allergic to these or just doesn't like it).

Time:
There is no Golden Rule as to the duration of a Reiki Treatment. Reiki is an „intelligent" energy. And the

body will take only as much as it needs, the rest will go elsewhere. So you cannot overdo it.

If you are treating a family member or a friend you should just rely on your intuition. So one session may be 80 minutes long, the next one only 30 minutes – just as needed.

But if you take money for a treatment the session should take at least one hour, unless you expressly offer and get paid for a „short treatment".

The Treatment Itself

As already pointed out, what follows are recommendations only, nothing is mandatory.

You could just put your hands on the recipient, let your intuition guide you and let the energy flow. And in a case of emergency you should never hesitate to do just that!

But especially as a beginner you may feel a little insecure. So this is the standard ritual:

The recipient lies down with his clothes still on (except for the shoes), and you cover him up with a light blanket unless the weather is extremely hot. When he starts relaxing the body functions slow down, so even if he felt warm before he might get cold.

Even though you will sometimes read it differently it is not necessary for the recipient to take off metal items such as wedding rings, watches etc.. But glasses would be disturbing during the treatment and should be put aside in a safe place. The same applies to big barrettes and other large embellishments.

The practitioner washes his hands. This is a ritual cleansing, your hands should be clean anyway, but it helps to start the energy flow.

You can say a little prayer if you want before starting the treatment, but this is not mandatory.

The actual treatment starts by „Smoothing out the aura": You run your leading hand 3 times counter-clockwise from head to toe and back 10 to 15 cm above the body of the recipient. This is the first contact you make with the energy field of the recipient. You can compare this to ringing the doorbell when you visit somebody. Just as you wouldn't just get into the house without announcing yourself, you announce yourself when you do Reiki by „Smoothing out the aura".

Then you lightly put your hands on the recipient's body and let the Reiki energy flow into his body.

As to the hand positions please refer to the photos in the next chapter.

When I started offering professional sessions I used to treat my clients from both sides, the front and the back. So I had to make them turn over after half of the session. However by that time most of them were in a deep trance or even fast asleep.

At a certain point I decided it doesn't really make sense to wake them up during the session! The Reiki energy flows directly into their energy system which circulates around their body, so it reaches their back anyway.

Therefore today I don't apply Reiki on the back anymore, unless the client asks for it – which hardly ever happens.

Instead of holding the 20 „official" positions which are usually held for 3 minutes each I'm using the 10 front positions only, to which I've added a few new ones (which actually mirror the ones on the back). In the next chapter I will show you both the official as well as my way, so you can decide for yourself how you prefer to do it.

As already said: These are just recommendations anyway. Feel free to skip positions - or add your own ones - just as you feel it's right! I always encourage my students to trust their own intuition. There are no „wrong" positions.

However there's one exception: If you know that somebody suffers from a medical condition it's safer to avoid the respective area, as a direct application of Reiki may be experienced as unpleasant.

For example someone with a heart disease shouldn't be treated directly over the heart, and if somebody suffers from epilepsy you must definitely leave out all head positions.

Pregnant women should better not be treated over their womb. Reiki cannot do harm and it won't cause a miscarriage as some people fear. But the baby is an individual with a free will. And you cannot ask if he or she likes having Reiki applied directly on them. Treat the mother's legs and arms instead!

Most clients experience a Reiki treatment as

something that's extremely nice, giving them a warm, cozy, relaxing feeling.

But there's always an exception to the rule. And just as not everybody likes to have a massage or go to to the hairdresser's, even though most people LOVE that, there are some people who don't like to receive Reiki.

If it is so, there's not much you can do. Always respect the client's free will and immediately take your hands off them if they ask you to stop. No discussion about that! However Distance Reiki might be an alternative for these clients if they still want to receive Reiki as the effects are more gentle.

It may also happen that a client dislikes just a specific hand position. When a lot of energy is set into motion, warmth develops. This is a typical effect during a Reiki session. But in some cases the heat can be quite extreme, and that may feel unpleasant for the recipient. For example it might cause a feeling of tightness in the chest area, or dizziness in the head.

So always encourage your clients to speak up if anything feels uncomfortable for them. They don't have to stand it – you can always skip a position, and maybe just hold another one a bit longer to make up for the time.

To finish the treatment „smoothe out the aura" again, 3 times counter-clockwise as described before.

Then, in order to reactivate the energy flow, you

position your left hand about 10 to 15 cm above the client's feet, holding it as if you wanted to perform a karate chop on him (which – of course – you are not going to do). Then quickly move that same hand towards his head, but without touching him. It should be a fast long movement along his body line, literally giving the energy in his aura a push to encourage it's flow.

There's something else that you need to know: Reiki cannot do harm, but just like people who are treated with Homeopathy some clients might experience a so-called „Primary Aggravation" over the following days.

This can even happen to apparently healthy clients, who sometimes may experience headaches or the return of old symptoms. Even though this may be causing them concern it's a positive sign, as it proves that Reiki starts working on them!

So you'd better let your clients know that this COULD but doesn't have to happen, and that nothing's wrong if it does.

It would be a pity if someone got worried and stopped the treatment, instead of just allowing what happens. If he gives the energy a chance it will bring up all old unresolved issues that need to be dealt with, so they can finally heal and be released once and for all!

The Hand Positions

The following photos show the 20 officially recommended hand positions of the Usui Reiki System of Natural Healing according to Dr. Hayashi.

A big Thank You goes to my husband Peter who took these photos as well as to our lovely model Larysa.

Provided you are right-handed always have the client lying on his back in front of you with his head to your right and his feet to your left (or his head to your left if you're left- handed).

After washing your hands first „smoothe out the client's aura". As I can't provide a picture here I'm going to describe this process once again in a slightly different way (supposing you are right-handed): Let the back of your left hand slightly rest at the side of the client's hip, just to make a contact, whilst your right hand is slowly circling counter clockwise about 10 to 15 cm above his body. Stretch out so the circle you make covers the whole length and width of the recipient's body, and repeat the movement 3 times.

Then put your hands on the client's body – without too much pressure. Each of the 20 positions should be held for 3 minutes, so a complete treatment takes exactly one hour.

Position 1

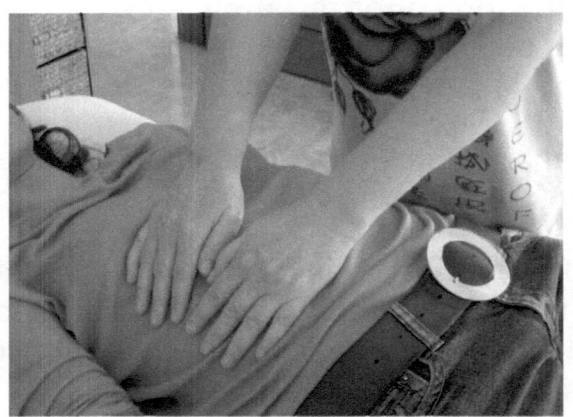

Position 2

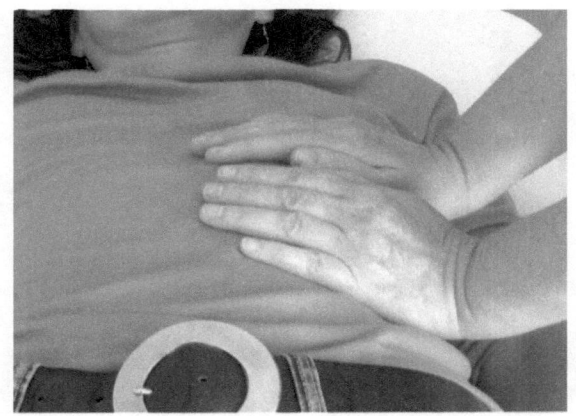

Position 3

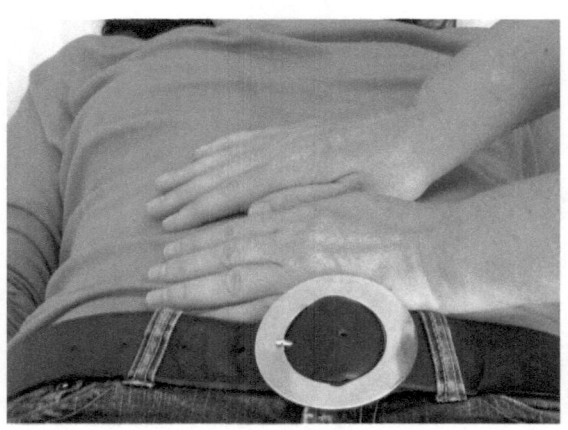

Position 4

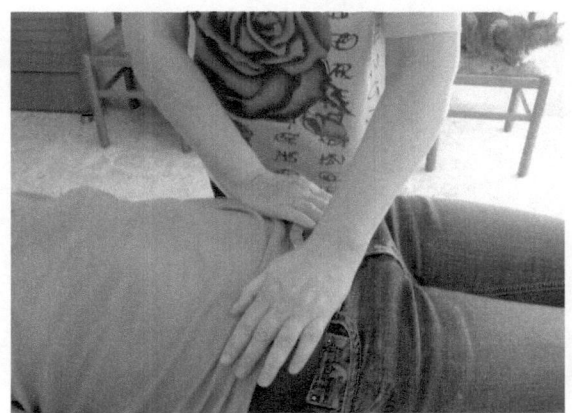

Position 5

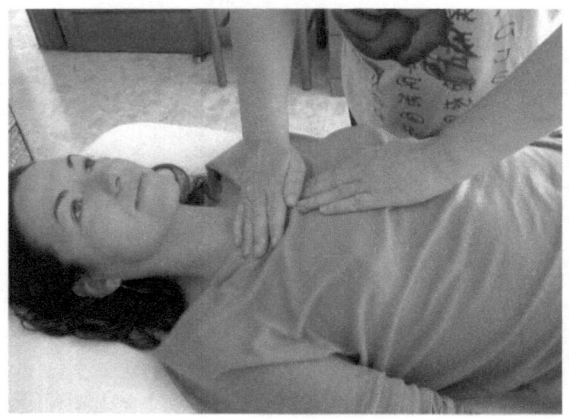

Position 6

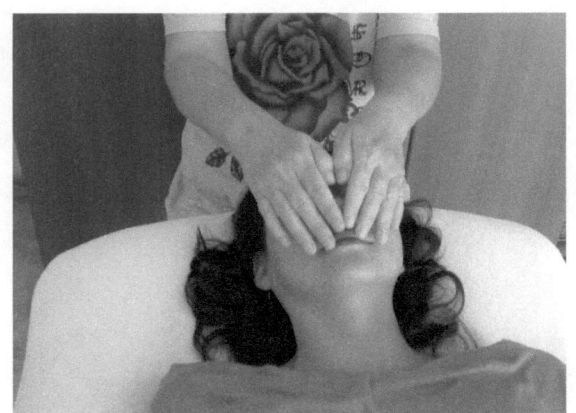

Position 7

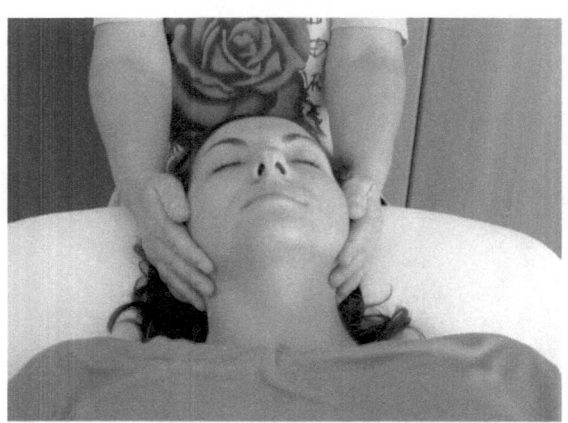

Position 8

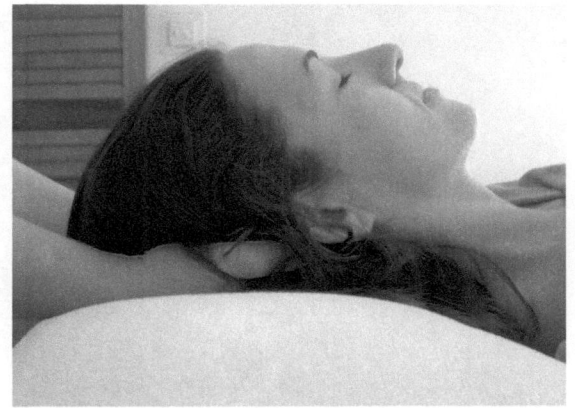

Position 9

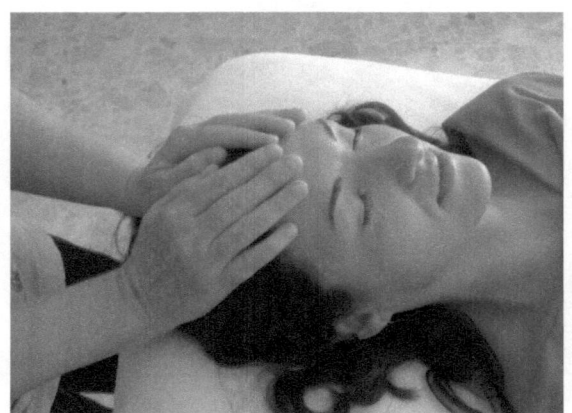

Position 10

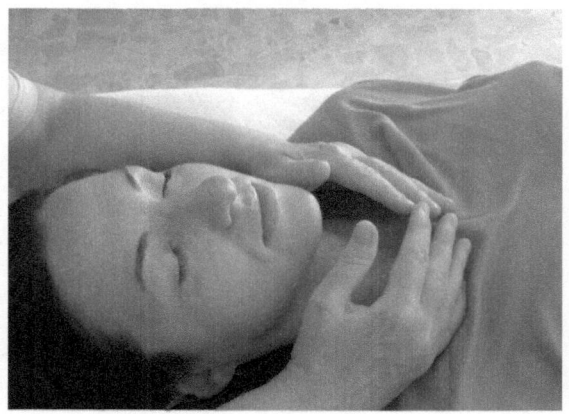

Position 11

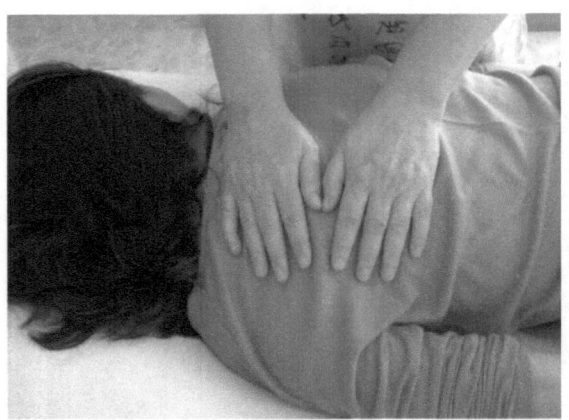

Position 12

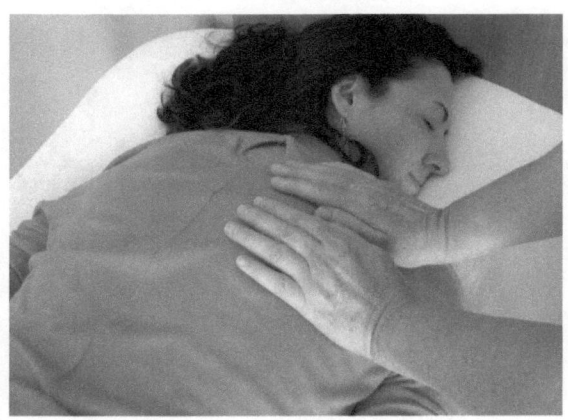

Position 13

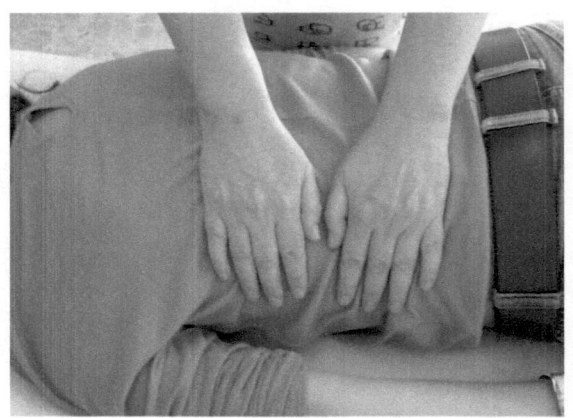

Position 14

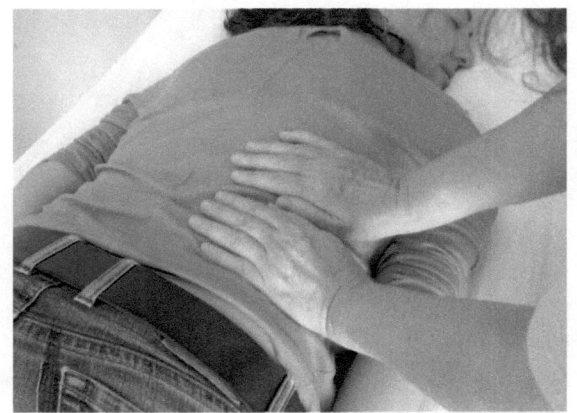

Position 15

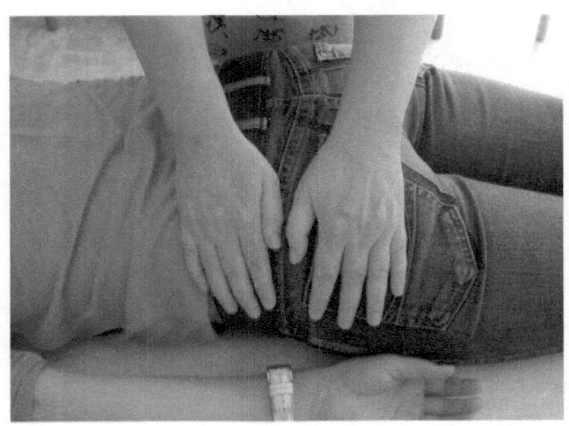

Position 16

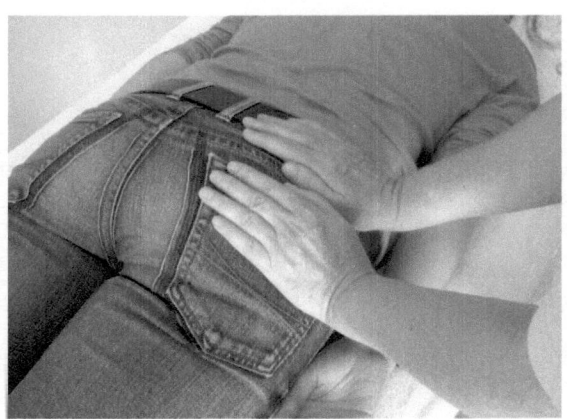

Position 17

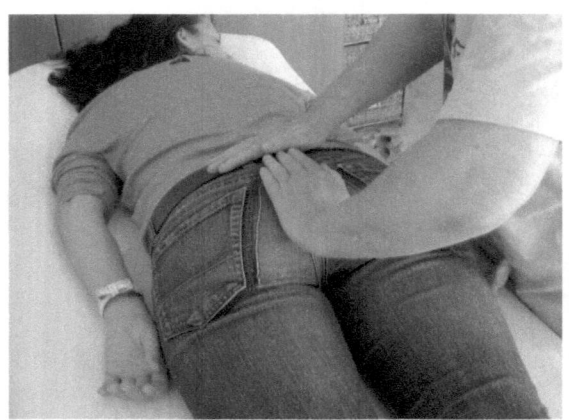

Position 18

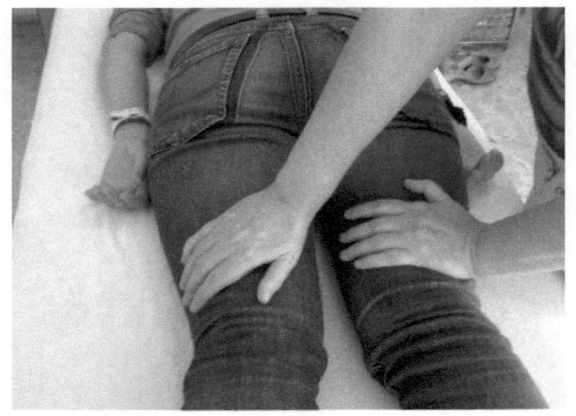

Position 19

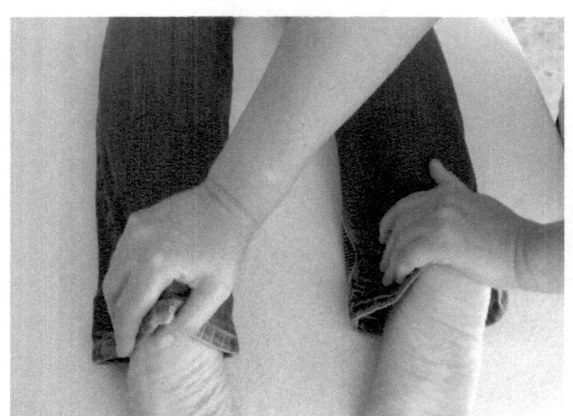

Position 20

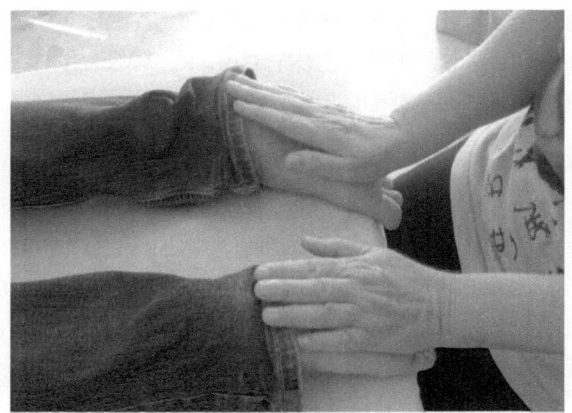

This is the last one of the „official" hand positions.

You finish off the treatment by „smoothing out the aura" once again and then giving the energy of the client a push as described above.

That ends the session.

As already mentioned I personally don't make the client turn over after half the session. Positions 1 to 10 remain the same, but then I'm using 5 extra positions on the face side for a total of 15.

To make up for the lost time due to the missing 5 positions I'm holding each of my 15 positions for a minimum of 4 minutes instead of the usual 3.

Reiki can easily be combined with other healing techniques, for example visualization and prayer. I'm usually doing this when holding the head positions, because then I'm sitting and can easily relax. I then visualize the Master Symbol, coming down on us in 3-dimensional form until it covers both the whole treatment bench and myself.

I'm also using Ho'oponopono, an old Hawaiian Healing Technique.

That's why I normally hold the head positions even a bit longer. In total my sessions are never shorter than 65 minutes, and often more if I feel the client really needs a boost.

Let me explain in a few words what Ho'oponopono is:

The basic concept of this Healing Technique is that we are the creators of our reality. But other than the usual „Law of Attraction" theories this includes not only our own lives but what happens to others too. So even if it's somebody else who is sick or has a problem, we still have co-created this. Once we know about it, it's in our reality, and that means we are responsible for it.

Please don't get me wrong, being responsible does not mean being guilty. Most of the time we create unconsciously anyway. However, as something in ourselves has contributed to this problem that the other person has, it's our responsibility to change it, and we can only change the outcome if we heal that part within us which has co-created it. And as we have no idea what we did in the first place, this can only be solved by presenting the matter to the Divine for help.

So after saying an introductory prayer we keep repeating the following Mantra, over and over, addressed to the Divine: „I'm sorry (meaning: sorry for contributing to this problem), please forgive me (meaning: please heal it), thank you (showing trust that your prayer will be answered), I love you!"...

If you want to know more about Ho'oponopono, I recommend you get the book „**Zero Limits" by Dr. Joe Vitale** (also available as an Audio-Book). It's an interesting read, and as strange as it may seem, this technique is very effective and makes the Reiki sessions even more powerful!

Now here are my 5 Extra-Positions:

My Position 11

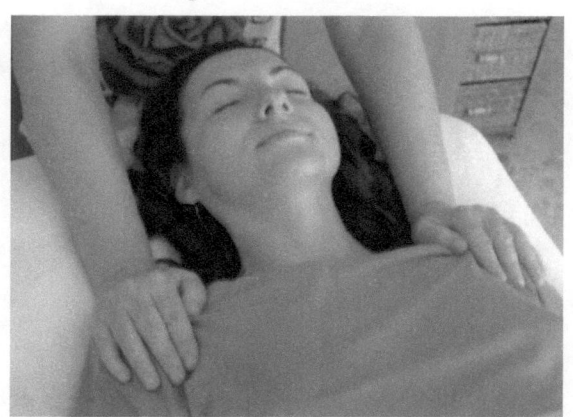

My Position 12

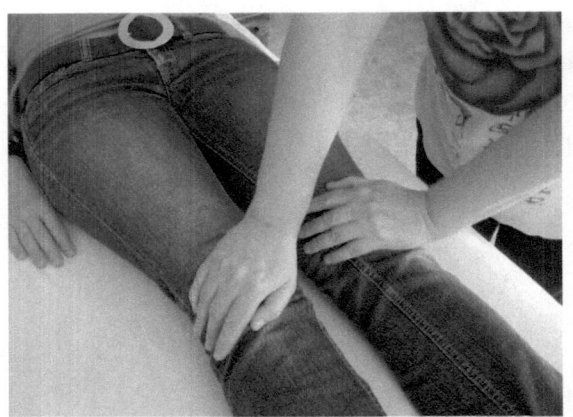

My Position 13

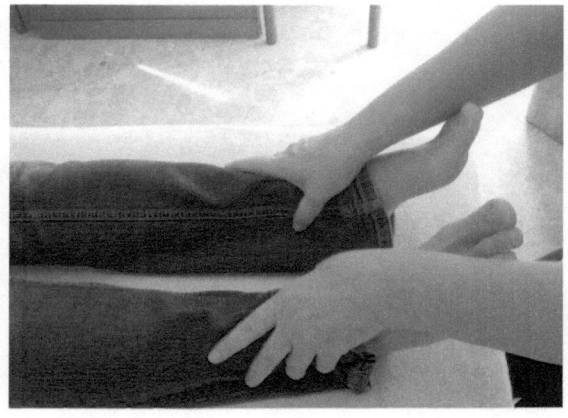

My Position 14

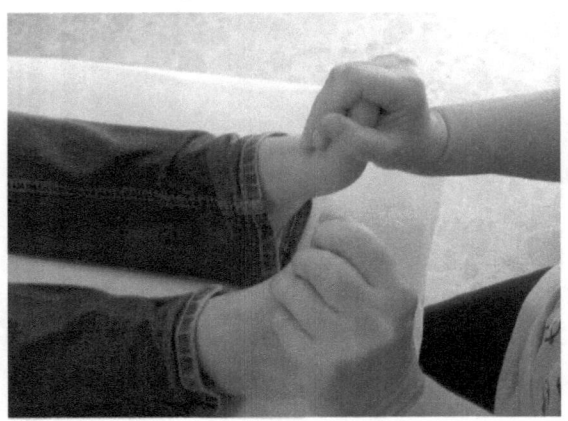

My Position 15

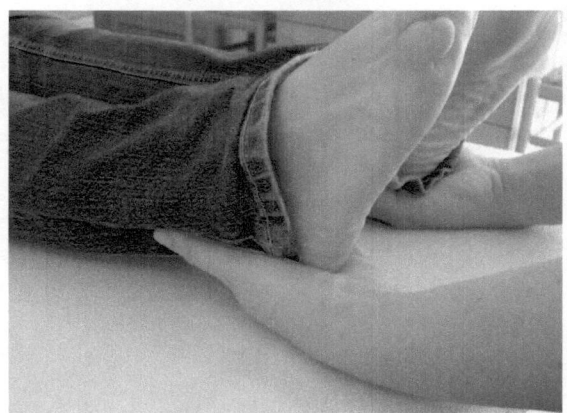

Once again: To finish the treatment „smoothe out the aura" 3 times and then give the client's energy a push as already described.

By the way, here's proof that many animals like Reiki a lot: Our beautiful cat Minku insisted on helping with the fotos!

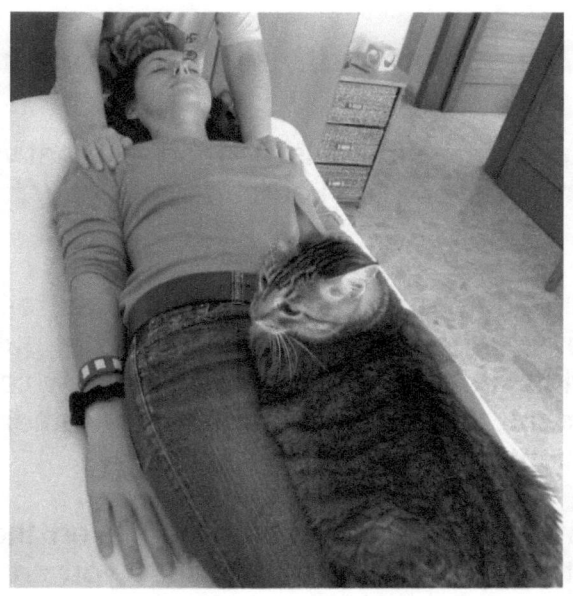

I'm really lucky that most of my clients love cats and don't mind his presence during the sessions, because he's giving me a hard time whenever I have to remove him from the treatment room ...

Quick Treatment (with the recipient sitting)

The following treatment is a good alternative to the regular treatment which you can use if you don't have a bench.

But as already mentioned it's not quite as relaxing for the recipient who has to sit. You also get quite close to him whilst holding the lower positions, which is why I recommend this for friends and family rather than for paying clients.

The treatment itself is very intense even though it's only 15 to 20 minutes long, because you are treating the recipient from the front and the back at the same time.

What you need is 2 normal chairs without armrests.

The recipient sits down on one of them with the backrest on his left bodyside, so you have free access to his back and right bodyside. He can lean with his left side against the backrest and should relax as good as possible.

Put the second chair somewhere on his right – this one is meant for you to use when you get to the lower positions.

You start by approaching the recipient from the back. „Smoothe out" his aura from the top down to the bottom using both hands, 3 times. Then lightly put your hands on his shoulders. This gesture is just meant to make a first contact, so you can immediately proceed to the first position.

The positions themselves are very easy to keep in mind, because they follow the location of the Chakras from top to bottom.

So the first position is on top of the recipient's head. Rest both of your hands there, still standing behind him. Hold this position for about 2 minutes or so.

Now move over to the recipient's right body side. Put your right hand on his forehead where the third eye is located, and the left hand over the medulla, on the back of his head. Again hold for about 2 minutes.

The next hand position is your right hand over the throat and your left hand in the neck. Make sure not to choke your patient while you hold this position for 2 minutes!

Then place your right hand over the recipient's heart and the other one between the bladebones for another 2 minutes.

The positions that follow are by far more comfortable for you to hold if you sit too, so pull your chair close to you now and sit down.

Place your right hand on the solar plexus of the recipient and the left hand on his kidney area, and again hold for 2 minutes.

Please note: Should you ever experience the

situation that you have to take care of a person who's in shock, this is the ideal emergency position!

First Aid guides recommend to place shock-patients in a lying position, but with the torso a bit upwards, and to keep them warm. And it's extremely important to have someone stay near them, constantly speaking to them in a soft and calming voice, in order to make sure that they don't jump up and run away (and then probably collapse somewhere).

Holding someone in this position you can attend to them and at the same time provide them with lots of healing Reiki energy! The solar plexus area is where we store our energy reserves, and the kidneys belong to our most delicate vital organs.

The next position is your right hand just below the recipient's bellybutton, and the other one on his lower back. You hold this one for ca. 2 minutes also.

For the last position put your right hand above the pubic area (you'd better not touch the recipient there unless you're VERY close ... but the Reiki energy is going to go where it's needed anyway) and the other one over the tailbone.

That's the last one of the „official" positions. But I always like to include the knees, as usually they really need it. They are doing a hard job for most people!

When you're done get up and stand behind the

recipient's back again. Repeat the „smoothing out" of the aura 3 times with both hands, then reactivate the client's energy field by quickly moving your left hand up from bottom to top with your palm pointing upwards.

Treating Yourself

Treating yourself with Reiki is very easy.

You don't have to say any prayers or need any magic rituals. All you have to do is decide that you could use a little Reiki and put your hands on your body. Reiki is going to flow automatically.

I personally love to give Reiki to myself while watching TV or listening to some music. I either place one hand on my heart and the other one on my solar plexus, or one hand on the solar plexus and the other one just below the bellybutton.
You can even treat yourself with Reiki when you are in public, without anybody having to notice. Just let one or both of your hands rest anywhere on your body, a thigh for example, and allow the energy to flow. Reiki will feed your energy field, which circulates through and around your body, so it's definitely going to reach the parts of your body where you need it the most.

If you're having a long day on the computer, it's also very nice to take a short break and put the palms of your hands over your eyes, so the eye muscles can completely relax in darkness. Even if you're not a Reiki practitioner it's highly recommended to practice this from time to time! But letting Reiki flow while you do it makes it even more effective.

So as you see there are quite a few possibilities to provide yourself with Reiki throughout the day. However sometimes you may feel that you want more and decide to treat yourself with a complete session.

Then you proceed like this:

First prepare the room. Make sure that you won't be disturbed for awhile, and don't forget to switch off your mobile phone or put it on mute!

Maybe you want to put on some soothing music, light a candle or evaporate a relaxing scent as you would do for a client – that's completely up to you. You may also combine the treatment with any other healing technique you like, such as (guided) meditation, affirmations or visualization.

Either sit comfortably or lie down (I personally prefer to lie down - but then sometimes I don't carry it through till the end because I fall asleep ...)

Hold each hand position as long as you like.

You start by putting the palms of your hands over your eyes.

Then place the palms of your hands right above your ears with the fingers pointing towards the crown of your head.

The next position is both hands on the back of your head, one of them placed directly on the medulla and the other one right above. But if you prefer you can also place the upper hand on the crown of your head instead. I personally find this more comfortable, especially when sitting, and you cover 2 Chakras at the same time. Just try it out for yourself. As I said:

There are no „wrong" positions, so whatever feels good for you is fine!

The following position is not an „official" one, so you can skip this if you want. But I love it – especially during the cold season. It works extremely well when you have a sore throat. Place your right hand on the right side of your throat and the left one on the left and then let your wrists touch in the middle. With the heat that's developing once Reiki flows it feels like there is a warm scarf lying around your neck, and that's a very comforting and soothing feeling!

The next „official" position would be one hand below your throat and one hand on your heart.

Then continue by putting one hand on your solar plexus and the other one right below your bellybutton.

The position that concludes the „official" positions for a self-treatment is both hands on your lower abdomen, with your hands building a „V".

As you may have noticed, these positions cover all the Chakras from top to bottom.

If you're sitting you can of course include the knees in the session, and maybe even your feet.

You should never cross your hands, as that would disturb the energy flow. But for most positions you can choose freely which one of your hands you position where. If for example it's one hand below the throat, one hand on the heart area, you can either put your right hand below the throat and your left over the heart, or do it the other way round. You may notice that the flow is a little stronger in your leading hand. But don't think too much about this. You will instinctively do it right. And if you are insecure, you can always switch hands after awhile.

Of course it's not necessary to „smoothe out the aura" when you're treating yourself. I've compared this to ringing the doorbell before entering someone else's house. But for your own house you've got a key, so there's no need to ring the bell!

Balancing the Chakras

If you're like me you are probably going to do a little research about Reiki on the internet, and sooner or later you will come across a special technique for balancing the Chakras using Reiki.

This method intentionally intrudes the client's energy system by aiming at making all the Chakras equally strong.

You put your hands about 10 cm above two Chakras, let's say the Root and the Heart Chakra, and feed them with energy until they feel the same. Then you equalize the Sacral and the Heart Chakra and so on, until they are all the same.

This technique is NOT part of the Usui System of Natural Healing.

As you may have noticed, the „official" hand positions as well as the ones I recommend here cover all the Chakras plus a few extra areas. So the Chakras are opened and balanced automatically during a session, and there's nothing more that needs to be done. You just provide the energy and allow every individual Chakra to take as much of it as is needed.

To me the new technique described above is dangerous, and the reason lies in the intention.

Every Chakra has it's own individual frequency, so who knows if it's beneficial for the client to make them all equal? Also - as you can see on the Chart that I provided - the Chakras are not only associated to specific body parts, but also to issues we may deal with in our lives. In total the way that our Chakras relate to each other make part of our personality.

And even with all Chakras open and fully functional, it's completely normal that some of them may be a little stronger than the others, whilst another one may not be quite as strong. That's part of our individuality!

Do we really want to be all the same?

Therefore in my opinion it's better not to use this technique. I hope this makes sense to you too.

The 21-day Purification Phase

After each attunement there is a so-called 21-day Purification Phase. Of course the phase doesn't have to last for 21 days exactly, it may take you few days more or less to get through it.

Psychologists agree that normally it takes 21 days to get used to changes and form a new habit, the mentioned time span may refer to that.

Anyway, body and mind have to deal with very strong energies. Changes will be initiated that are more or less perceptible, and old unresolved stuff may come up in order to finally heal and be released.

So if you suffer from mood swings and feel like crying sometimes this is absolutely normal.

At the same time the body will be purified. So you might sweat more than you usually do, or maybe you will have to go to the restroom more frequently.

You should help yourself by drinking a lot of water and eating balanced healthy food. Of course you can have meat, if you're not a vegetarian, but it should be lean if possible and not the fatty stuff.

This phase is the reason why I recommend you should wait **at least 3 weeks** before you move on to the next Reiki Degree.

Even if you feel ready for it, these are very strong

energies that shouldn't be underestimated! And being attuned to two or even more Reiki Degrees at the same time may just be more that you can handle.

Last but not least

This concludes my little book.

I hope that you found it helpful.

If you have further questions, please feel free to contact me under my email address reikibooks@gmail.com

I'd be happy to hear from you!

Also if you liked my book I'd be grateful if you'd give it a 4 or 5-star review on Kindle!

Thanks for your interest, and all the best to you!

Love and light

Antje Seebohm

www.ingramcontent.com/pod-product-compliance
Lightning Source LLC
Chambersburg PA
CBHW022345290526
45786CB00014B/2500